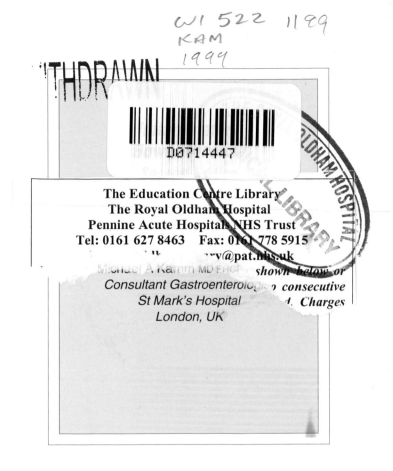

Michael A Kamm MD FRCP
Consultant Gastroenterologist
St Mark's Hospital
London, UK

MARTIN DUNITZ

Although every effort has been made to ensure that the drug doses and other information are presented accurately in this publication, the ultimate responsibility rests with the prescribing physician. Neither the publishers nor the author can be held responsible for errors or for any other consequences arising from the use of information contained herein.

© Martin Dunitz Ltd 1999

First published in the United Kingdom
in 1996 by
Martin Dunitz Ltd
The Livery House
7– 9 Pratt Street
London NW1 0AE

A CIP record for this book is available from the British Library.

ISBN 1-85317-641-9

Printed and bound in Spain by Cayfosa

Contents

Introduction

This book is a clinician's guide to the commonest inflammatory bowel diseases – ulcerative colitis and Crohn's disease – as well as related conditions such as 'pouchitis' and microscopic colitis. It is not intended to be an exhaustive text, but rather to provide:

- A clinical guide to **proven management regimes**
- An overview of **recent developments** in the fields of epidemiology, genetics, immune mechanisms, natural history of disease, prognosis and cancer risk
- A guide to **new therapies** currently available and some likely to be important in the near future

There is a special emphasis on dealing with the questions that patients are likely to ask, such as:

- What causes this condition?
- Am I likely to pass it on to my children?
- Should I alter my diet?
- Should I be on a 'new' steroid with fewer side-effects?
- Are there new drugs which can prevent an urgent colectomy?
- What is the risk of the disease extending?
- What is the chance that I will require surgery?
- What is my risk of developing cancer?

Epidemiology

Inflammatory bowel disease is more common in Europe and North America than in tropical Africa, South America, Asia and Japan. Differences in incidence between the North and South of Europe are smaller than previously reported. The prevalence of both conditions, especially Crohn's disease, appears to have risen over the last 40 years.

In Western populations the prevalence of ulcerative colitis is approximately 1 in 1000, and of Crohn's disease 1 in 1500 of the population

- The incidence of Crohn's disease and ulcerative colitis is greatest in early adult life, with a second smaller peak of ulcerative colitis in the elderly
- Both conditions are slightly more common in women than men
- The prevalence is the same in different social classes
- Black people are affected less often than white people in North America
- Jewish people living or born outside Israel have increased susceptibility to both Crohn's disease and ulcerative colitis, suggesting an aetiological mix of environmental and genetic factors

---

Aetiology

Environmental factors

Smoking

Smoking confers protection against the development of ulcerative colitis, with the lowest incidence in smokers, intermediate incidence in ex-smokers, and highest incidence in non-smokers. The reverse is true for Crohn's disease, in which smoking increases the risk of developing the disease and doubles the risk of postoperative recurrence.

Oral contraceptives

There may be a slight association between oral contraceptive use and the development of Crohn's disease. This is insufficient to deny a patient the oral contraceptive, unless they have had previous venothrombotic disease or have a risk of poor absorption because of diarrhoea or a short small intestine.

Infective agents

Despite much effort, incontrovertible evidence of an infective cause for ulcerative colitis or Crohn's disease has not emerged.

Measles virus has been suggested as a possible cause of Crohn's disease, based on:

- Epidemiological evidence of a disease association with vaccination programmes
- A possible increased incidence of Crohn's disease in offspring after maternal measles infection during pregnancy
- Tissue studies suggesting the presence of measles virus in a higher than expected proportion of patients with Crohn's disease

A definitive relationship between this virus and Crohn's disease remains to be established.

Mycobacterium paratuberculosis has also been put forward as a possible cause of Crohn's disease, because this organism:

- Causes a similar disease affecting the small intestine in cattle (Johne's disease)
- Can be found in Crohn's disease tissue, although it can also be isolated in other intestinal conditions
- Can be found in milk

However, trials of antituberculous therapy have not yielded a cure in Crohn's disease.

Genetic factors

The genetic contribution to the aetiology of both Crohn's disease and ulcerative colitis is polygenic in pattern rather than simple Mendelian. Data from the Swedish twin registry have shown a proband concordance rate among monozygotic twins of 6% for ulcerative colitis and 58% for Crohn's disease, suggesting a stronger genetic influence in Crohn's disease. It is most likely that a large number of genes contribute to a predisposition to inflammatory bowel disease (IBD), and more of these genes are present in patients who develop Crohn's disease.

Susceptibility loci on chromosomes 16, 12, 7, and 3 have been found for inflammatory bowel disease, but these are unlikely to be the only genetic determinants that confer susceptibility to such disorders. There is currently a lack of consistency between linkage studies in different populations, further suggesting that the genetic determinants of such disorders are complex

Risk within families (Table 1)

The risk of a patient with Crohn's disease having an affected first degree relative (parent, sibling or child) is about 10 times the population risk. When considering the extended family, 20–30% of patients have a positive family history of IBD, although the affected relative(s) often have the other disease. Spouses of patients with IBD have a low risk of developing IBD.

Risk of	Sibling/parent having IBD	Child developing IBD
Patient with UC	1–3%	1–3%
Patient with CD	3–8%	1–2%

Table 1
Risk of family members having or developing IBD.

Genetic markers

A particular subgroup of perinuclear antineutrophil cytoplasmic antibodies (P-ANCA) is seen in 50–80% of patients with ulcerative colitis, and is also commonly seen in patients with IBD and sclerosing cholangitis. They are found in 10–20% of patients with Crohn's disease. ANCA are unlikely to contribute to the pathogenesis of IBD but may have particular use as a marker of underlying immunological disturbance that is genetically determined.

Genetic disease associations

Patients with ulcerative colitis and Crohn's disease have an increased incidence of ankylosing spondylitis, and 90% or more patients with IBD and ankylosing spondylitis are HLA-B27 positive.

Neither ulcerative colitis nor Crohn's disease are consistently associated with HLA-A, HLA-B, or HLA-DR antigens, apart from minor associations in some populations.

Enteric bacteria

Research suggests that an abnormal immune response to common enteric bacteria and yeasts, combined with genetic susceptibility, causes or contributes to the inflammatory process.

Proliferation of peripheral and lamina propria T lymphocytes to bacterial, mycobacterial, and fungal antigens has been shown. Titres of mucosal IgG antibodies are higher in patients with Crohn's disease and ulcerative colitis than in controls, and some of these antibodies are directed against cytoplasmic antigens of commensal bacterial flora. Mucosal lymphocytes from healthy individuals are tolerant of their own bacterial flora, whereas lymphocytes from patients with inflammatory bowel disease proliferate when cocultured with their own bacterial antigens.

Serum antibodies and proliferative lymphocyte responses to *Saccharomyces cerevisiae* (bakers and brewers yeast) are significantly increased in patients with Crohn's disease, when compared to patients with ulcerative colitis or healthy controls.

Amongst the most compelling evidence implicating exogenous antigens in Crohn's disease is that of persistent CD4$^+$ cell clones in the peripheral blood of patients with Crohn's disease. These T-cell clones are shared in patients with similar HLA types, suggesting a link between exogenous antigens and the patient's genetic background in T-cell clonal expansion which leads to mucosal damage.

Inflammatory bowel disease has not been observed in animals with a genetically induced absence of single cytokines, such as IL-2 and IL-10, if the gut is kept sterile. Inflammation occurs rapidly when common enteric flora are introduced.

Mechanisms of inflammation

In inflammatory bowel disease a wide diversity of immunological changes occur, including altered populations of inflammatory cells and the activation of a range of inflammatory pathways (Figure 1).

The gut mucosa has effective functional and anatomical immune compartments. The most specialized sites for antigen processing are the Peyer's patches located in the ileum, consisting of both B and T cells. When a lumenal antigen crosses the epithelial layer, specialized cells (dendritic cells and macrophages) process the antigen and present it to T cells. This interaction promotes the proliferation of antigen-specific B and T cells. B cells secrete immunoglobulins, predominantly IgA, while the T cells undergo clonal proliferation in the mesenteric lymph nodes. These activated and replicated cells migrate back to the lamina propria, where an effector response occurs, resulting in inflammation. This process involves special proteins – cytokines – which are secreted by the T cells, macrophages, and epithelial cells.

'Activated' T lymphoctyes (helper cells and cytotoxic cells) are normally found in the gut wall. However, in inflammatory bowel disease the normal regulation of their activity is disturbed.

Process of lymphoid cell priming and migration to lamina propria

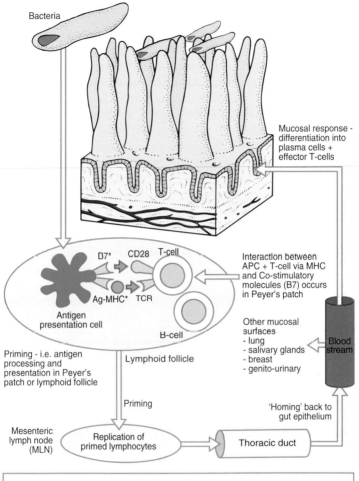

Bacteria

Mucosal response - differentiation into plasma cells + effector T-cells

B7* CD28 T-cell

Ag-MHC* TCR

Antigen presentation cell

B-cell

Interaction between APC + T-cell via MHC and Co-stimulatory molecules (B7) occurs in Peyer's patch

Priming - i.e. antigen processing and presentation in Peyer's patch or lymphoid follicle

Lymphoid follicle

Other mucosal surfaces
- lung
- salivary glands
- breast
- genito-urinary

Blood stream

Priming

Mesenteric lymph node (MLN)

Replication of primed lymphocytes

Thoracic duct

'Homing' back to gut epithelium

*B7 + MHC are molecules involved in antigen presentation to the T-cell
MHC - TCR interaction necessary for antigen-specific response by naive T-cell
B7 - CD28 interaction with co-stimulating molecules necessary for optimal activation of T-cell in addition to MHC - TCR, otherwise tolerance can develop.

Figure 1
Inflammatory mechanisms in inflammatory bowel disease. With thanks to Dr Steven Mann.

Whether this is due to a normal specific response to an unknown antigen, or due to impaired self-regulation of the response to normal antigens, is unknown.

Activation of mucosal inflammatory cells also leads to the production of a large number of inflammatory mediators, which are at least partly responsible for the tissue damage observed in these conditions. These mediators include prostaglandins, leukotrienes, platelet activating factor, thromboxanes, oxygen radicals, proteases, and cytokines. For some of these inflammatory mediators, their suppression leads to activation of other pathways which allow inflammation to continue. Other substances, such as tumour necrosis factor (TNF), have a central role and suppression may lead to diminished inflammation. Cytokines responsible for tissue repair are also produced in increased amounts in these disorders.

Leukotrienes

Leukotriene B4 (LTB4) is a major proinflammatory mediator produced by neutrophils, macrophages, and mast cells. It is produced from the substrate arachidonic acid via the 5-lipoxygenase pathway. It amplifies the cascade that stimulates neutrophil function. Tissue concentrations of this mediator are high in inflamed bowel.

Platelet activating factor

Platelet activating factor (PAF) is a family of potent inflammatory mediator compounds produced by vascular endothelial cells, by activated neutrophils, and by macrophages, in response to stimulation by interleukin-1 and tumour necrosis factor. The effects of PAF include aggregation of platelets, degranulation of neutrophils, and changes in vascular permeability.

Cytokines

Cytokines are low molecular weight regulatory proteins produced by most cells in response to injury, infection or antigen challenge. Gut epithelial cells, together with intramucosal inflammatory cells, are capable of secreting a large range of cytokines. These cytokines mediate cell growth, repair, immune activity and motility. Some of the differences observed between patients with the same disease may be related to polymorphism in the genes controlling cytokine production.

Interleukins 1β, 2, 6 and 8, and interferon-gamma are pro-inflammatory cytokines, produced in increased amounts in Crohn's disease and ulcerative colitis. Tumour necrosis factor consists of a family of proinflammatory cytokines. Interleukins 4, 5, 10 and 13 are immunoregulatory and may have a pro-repair role.

Interleukin-1

This family consists of three structurally-related polypeptides – interleukin-1α (IL-1α), interleukin-1β (IL-1β) and interleukin-1–receptor antagonist (IL-1–RA). Increased production of IL-1 occurs in inflammatory bowel disease, either as part of the inflammatory or the defence process.

Interleukin-2

IL-2 is essential for the proliferation, differentiation and clonal expansion of T cells. IL-2 deficient mice develop inflammation similar to ulcerative colitis.

Tumour necrosis factor (TNF)

Tumour necrosis factor alpha (TNF-α) is a proinflammatory cytokine produced by mononuclear cells and activated T cells during active inflammatory bowel disease. It affects neutrophil adhesion, leucocyte recruitment and the modulation of other cytokines. TNF levels in faeces correlate with intestinal inflammatory activity. The genes controlling TNF production are within the central region of the major histocompatibility complex (MHC) on chromosome 6, further suggesting a possible central role for TNF in promoting inflammation.

Interferons

Interferons enhance macrophage activity, modulate the response of B and T cells to antigen stimulation, and potentiate the natural killer activity of lymphocytes.

Tissue metalloproteinases

The metalloproteinases constitute a family of enzymes whose main function is the degradation of the extracellular matrix. The tissue destruction that occurs in inflammatory bowel disease involves these enzymes, and the effects of proinflammatory cytokines such as tumor necrosis factor alpha appear to be mediated at least in part through the activation of these metalloproteinase enzymes.

Experimental models of inflammation

Different experimental models are useful for studying different aspects of inflammatory bowel disease, such as:

- Genetic and environmental factors
- Immune mechanisms
- Response to drug healing
- Development of cancer

In experimental animals inflammation can be induced using immune complexes, formalin, acid, indomethacin, carrageenin and dextran sulphate sodium.

To study ankylosing spondylitis and associated enteropathies, transgenic rats expressing HLA-B27 and B2 microglobulin genes have been produced. Some develop spontaneous colitis, arthritis and psoriasis-like skin disease. Expression of B27, which may be recognized by T cells, is limited to lymphoid tissue in the gut and not epithelial cells.

Chronic recurrent colitis occurs spontaneously in cotton-top tamarins held in captivity. With increasing age these monkeys with colitis also have a high incidence of colonic adenocarcinoma. The colitis, and development of cancer after a prolonged period of disease on the background of dysplasia, bears a remarkable similarity to human disease.

IL-2 is an important regulatory cytokine which promotes growth and expansion of T cells, differentiation of B cells, and macrophage activation. Of mice bred to be homozygous for a disrupted IL-2 gene, those that survive develop a pancolitis. They have a high level of activated T and B cells, and expression of major histocompatibility complex class II antigens on the colonic epithelium.

IL-10 is also an important regulatory cytokine produced by T cells, certain B cells and macrophages. IL-10 is a potent inhibitor of macrophages and the Th1-cell subset. IL-10 homozygous gene knockout mice develop chronic inflammatory bowel disease affecting the whole gut. Bacterial colonization is necessary for disease expression, which is thought to be caused by an enhanced Th1 response to enteric bacteria. Administration of IL-10 effectively treats the disease.

Ulcerative colitis and Crohn's disease differ in their epidemiology, clinical manifestations, regions of affected intestine, gut pathology, nature of the immune reaction and response to treatment. They probably also differ in their aetiology (see pages 3–7).

Ulcerative colitis

Symptoms

The main symptoms are:

- Rectal bleeding
- Passage of mucus
- Diarrhoea
- Urgency
- Abdominal pain

In patients with limited proctitis the main complaint may only be the passage of blood and mucus, and urgency. Loose motions occur only in patients with more extensive large bowel inflammation. Cramping is the most common pain – this is associated with urgency, lasts only a few minutes, and is related to high pressure colonic contractions. Prolonged pain is usually only seen with more severe substantial colitis.

Anatomical extent

Ulcerative colitis extends for a variable distance from the lowermost rectum, just above the anal canal. Patients can therefore experience:

- Proctitis (rectum only inflamed)
- Left-sided colitis (distal to splenic flexure)
- Colitis extending from hepatic flexure ('substantial')
- Total colitis (whole colon inflamed, also known as 'extensive')

The extent of macroscopic involvement can progress or regress with time. If colonoscopic biopsies are taken from around the whole colon in patients with distal disease, inflammatory changes are often identified proximally. The selection of treatment, for example suppositories, enemas, or systemic drugs (see pages 46—51), can be based on the macroscopic extent. The risk of cancer also appears to relate to the macroscopic extent (see page 76).

Diagnosis

The anatomical extent and severity of inflammation should be determined. Initial sigmoidoscopy, either rigid or flexible, provides the likely diagnosis. It may also indicate anatomical extent, as well as providing the opportunity for mucosal biopsy. If there is limited proctitis the upper limit of inflammation will be visible, precluding the need for colonoscopy or X-rays.

If the upper limit of inflammation cannot be seen, it should be determined by colonoscopy or contrast studies. Colonoscopy should only be performed when the disease is mildly active, due to the increased risk of perforation in severely active disease.

If the anatomical extent needs to be determined at initial presentation with severe disease, in order to choose appropriate treatment, an 'instant' barium enema can be performed without bowel preparation (Figure 2).

Severe and fulminant colitis

Severe episodes of ulcerative colitis are characterized by:

- High bowel frequency (greater than eight per day)
- Abdominal pain and tenderness
- Marked blood loss

Fulminant colitis is characterized by systemic disturbance, such as:

- Tachycardia
- Fever
- Anaemia
- Malaise

The major concern in patients with severe or fulminant disease is **colonic dilatation and perforation.** Although mostly seen in severe episodes of total colitis, this can also occur in patients with severe left-sided disease. Warning signs are:

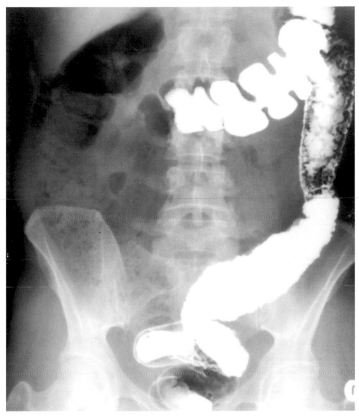

Figure 2
Unprepared 'instant' enema in a patient with acute ulcerative colitis. There is moderately severe ulceration involving the left colon. The transverse colon is also granular, suggesting at least mild inflammation. The right colon and caecum contain stool, suggesting that this part of the large bowel is not inflamed.

- Systemic toxicity (tachycardia, fever)
- Abdominal distension
- Tenderness to palpation and rebound

These signs can be masked in patients on steroids.

Patients should be closely monitored clinically and with sequential plain abdominal X-rays. Radiological signs of very severe disease include the presence of mucosal islands, which indicate destruction of mucosa with deep ulceration and separation of the lamina propria and mucosa from the muscularis propria, and dilatation. A colonic diameter of greater than 6.5 cm indicates toxic dilatation, provided that the mucosal outline is also irregular with loss of normal haustral markings. Perforation can also occur with a lesser diameter.

Recurrent episodes

Recurrent episodes tend to run 'true to form', with patients having the same extent of disease and responding to the same treatments. Occasionally the disease extends or an episode is more severe, demanding a change in therapy.

With new flare-ups it is important always to exclude infection by stool culture. If infection is present the colitis usually needs to be treated in addition to the enteric infection.

Crohn's disease

Symptoms

These depend on the distribution (Table 2) and severity of disease, together with the presence of complications.

The most common symptoms are:

> - Diarrhoea
> - Abdominal pain
> - Rectal bleeding
> - Anorexia
> - Weight loss

Site	Frequency
Extensive small bowel disease	5%
Ileum only	25%
Ileocaecal	40%
Colon only	25%
Miscellaneous (eg confined to anorectum, oral, gastric)	2%

Table 2
Distribution of Crohn's disease.

The main feature in patients with small bowel disease is pain. If this is mainly postprandial it may indicate partial intestinal obstruction. The main features in patients with colonic disease are diarrhoea and bleeding. Pain in patients with colonic disease is mainly related to defecation.

Physical examination

The main features to elicit are:

- Anaemia
- Oral ulceration
- Abdominal tenderness and masses
- Anal tags, fissure and fistulae

The most common causes of anaemia are chronic disease and chronic blood loss with iron deficiency. Malabsorption of haematinics is less common.

An important feature in children is growth retardation (see page 56). Children should have their height and weight recorded at each visit, and plotted on percentile charts

Pouchitis

Aetiology

The aetiology of pouchitis after colectomy and ileorectal anastomosis is unknown but it is likely to be a form of recurrent ulcerative colitis. The ileal mucosa of patients with previous ulcerative colitis appears to be susceptible to the effects of prolonged exposure to intestinal contents, especially enteric bacteria. The condition is rarely seen in patients having an ileoanal reservoir for familial polyposis coli, and is more common in patients who have had extraintestinal manifestations of their ulcerative colitis, such as sclerosing cholangitis.

Incidence

Non-specific inflammation of the ileal reservoir ('pouchitis') can result in symptoms identical to ulcerative colitis.

The incidence increases with time. About a third to a half of all ulcerative colitis patients will have experienced at least one episode of pouchitis 10 years after the pouch creation. Forty per cent of patients with pouchitis will have a single episode, with the remainder having at least one recurrence. Five per cent of all patients with a pouch will require chronic maintenance therapy ('chronic pouchitis').

Diagnosis

The diagnosis is based on a combination of:

- Symptoms, especially diarrhoea
- The endoscopic finding of inflammation
- Histological changes of **acute inflammation** (neutrophil infiltration and ulceration)

Histological changes of villous atrophy and the presence of a chronic inflammatory cell infiltrate are part of the normal colonic metaplasia that occurs after pouch creation, and are not signs of pouchitis.

Collagenous colitis/microscopic (lymphocytic) colitis

Collagenous colitis presents clinically as diarrhoea of unknown cause. About 80% of patients are women and it most commonly presents in middle age. The main features of collagenous colitis are:

- Chronically relapsing course
- Watery diarrhoea, sometimes large volumes (up to 2–3 litres/day)
- May be associated with abdominal pain, nausea and weight loss
- Secretory diarrhoea on osmotic stool testing
- Normal radiology and endoscopy of the small and large intestine

Associations

The following need to be actively investigated:

- Use of nonsteroidal anti-inflammatory drugs
- Coeliac disease
- Thyroid disease

The pathognomonic abnormality is **collagen deposition** beneath the subepithelial basement membrane, so that the thickness of the subepithelial band exceeds the normal upper limit of 10 μm (Figure 3). There is an associated **chronic inflammatory cell infiltrate**.

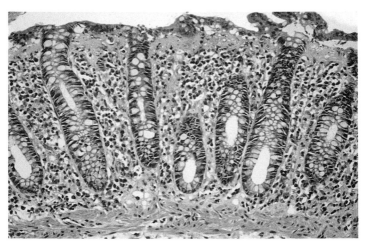

Figure 3
Collagenous colitis histology showing thickened subepithelial collagen plate and lamina propria inflammatory infiltrate.

There is an overlap of this condition with that of **microscopic colitis**, which presents with identical watery diarrhoea and macroscopically normal large bowel mucosa. Biopsies reveal an inflammatory lymphocytic infiltrate in the epithelium and lamina propria.

Microscopic polymorphonuclear inflammation

Some patients with diarrhoea and an endoscopically normal colon have acute (polymorph) inflammation on colonic biopsies, without subepithelial collagen thickening.

This condition is thought to be a microscopic form of ulcerative colitis or Crohn's disease. It usually responds to a 5-ASA drug, although rarely steroids are required. Some patients progress to macroscopic ulcerative colitis or Crohn's disease, sometimes after a number of years.

Extra-intestinal manifestations

Skin

Erythema nodosum and pyoderma gangrenosum occur in 2–10% of patients with IBD.

Erythema nodosum consists of raised painful swellings (most commonly on the shins) and usually reflects underlying intestinal inflammation. It usually responds to a course of oral steroids.

Pyoderma gangrenosum occurs in both ulcerative colitis and Crohn's disease. It occurs most commonly on the lower legs but may occur elsewhere, including around a stoma. It often starts as sterile fluid-filled blisters which soon ulcerate. It is harder to treat than erythema nodosum, and usually requires oral steroids. Occasionally, azathioprine is also necessary. Some patients will require a colectomy if the condition cannot be brought under control with drug therapy. Removing the colon and rectum in a patient with ulcerative colitis and severe unresponsive pyoderma will sometimes heal the pyoderma, but this is not universal. Sometimes, the pyoderma remains active (Figure 4).

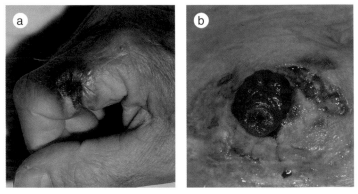

Figure 4
(a) Pyoderma gangrenosum on the hand of a patient with ulcerative colitis. His pyoderma resolved after he had a proctocolectomy and ileostomy.
(b) Peristomal pyoderma in a woman who had a colectomy for indeterminate colitis. The rectum was still present in situ.

Joints

Arthralgia and arthritis

Arthralgia of peripheral joints and the spine occur in most patients with IBD at some time in their illness, and most commonly are not associated with signs of joint inflammation or X-ray changes. Occasionally, effusions in large joints may occur.

There are several clinical patterns of joint involvement:

> - a large joint acute oligoarthropathy which can be associated with relapses of inflammatory bowel disease
> - a polyarthropathy involving peripheral joints, which appears to run a clinical course independent of inflammatory bowel disease activity
> - sacroileitis and ankylosing spondylitis in HLA-B27 positive patients with inflammatory bowel disease. The course of the joint disease is independent of the course of the gut inflammation

All three of these clinical patterns of arthropathy appear to have HLA associations that are genetically distinct.

Sometimes a nonsteroidal anti-inflammatory drug is required. Rarely, a short course of steroids is needed, although this only helps about half the patients.

Pouch-related arthritis
New joint symptoms can arise after proctocolectomy and pouch formation in patients with ulcerative colitis.

Femoral head necrosis
A rare but severe complication of steroid therapy involves the development of femoral head necrosis, which is presumed to relate to vascular infarction. The X-ray changes are typical. This complication means that the use of corticosteroids should be restricted to the minimum amount necessary in patients with inflammatory bowel disease, and that other immunosuppressives should be sought for long-term therapy.

Eyes

Anterior uveitis, episcleritis, and conjunctivitis all occur more commonly in patients with IBD. The eye symptoms may or may not parallel the intestinal activity.

Liver

Minor abnormalities of liver function tests occur in approximately 50% of patients with IBD. Fatty liver is the most common condition to occur in severe episodes of Crohn's disease or ulcerative colitis.

Pericholangitis, primary sclerosing cholangitis, and cholangiocarcinoma form part of the spectrum of primary sclerosing cholangitis, an inflammatory disorder involving the intra-hepatic and extra-hepatic biliary system. Endoscopic retrograde cholangiopancreatography (ERCP) allows a radiological diagnosis to be made. Associated abnormalities include inflammatory changes on liver biopsy and a cholestatic pattern on biochemical testing.

Amyloidosis

This is a rare complication of Crohn's disease that can involve all the main viscera, and which can lead to terminal hepatic or renal failure. It should be excluded in any patient with long-standing Crohn's disease who develops proteinuria.

Thromboembolic disease

Patients with IBD have a heightened intravascular coaguable state, related to an increased concentration of coagulation pathway factors and platelet count. Patients are at increased risk of perioperative thromboembolic disease, especially if they smoke, have been bed-bound, or have pelvic sepsis. These patients should have maximum prophylactic anticoagulation if surgery is required.

Clinical examination

The presence of extensive perianal fistulae and anal induration is more in keeping with Crohn's disease than ulcerative colitis. Patients with Crohn's disease are also more likely to have mouth ulcers.

Endoscopy

Rigid or flexible procto-sigmoidoscopy will establish the diagnosis of ulcerative colitis, or less commonly Crohn's proctitis. Mild inflammation may consist of erythema, or granularity with increased contact bleeding. The main features are ulceration, bleeding, and mucopus production.

Colonoscopy allows the pattern and severity of colonic and terminal ileum inflammation to be determined, and allows biopsies to be obtained. It should not be undertaken during acute or severe disease because of the increased risk of perforation. The presence of postinflammatory polyps ('pseudo-polyps') indicates previous severe inflammation.

If the inflammation is confluent, either condition may be present. If there are isolated aphthous ulcers with intervening normal mucosa, then Crohn's disease is most likely.

Differential diagnosis

Other conditions to consider if there is terminal ileal or colonic inflammation include:

- Tuberculosis
- Bacterial infection
- Yersinia — if the terminal ileum only is inflamed
- Parasitic infection including amoebiasis or schistosomiasis if the patient has visited, or comes from, an endemic area
- Bechet's disease if there are deep punched-out ulcers

Infection can also occur in patients with known IBD, and should be excluded by routine stool culture during new acute episodes of diarrhoeal illness.

If there is only proctitis, consider:

- Gonococcus (sexually transmitted; usually much mucopus — culture)
- Chlamydia (sexually transmitted — culture)
- In immunocompromised or HIV-infected patients — cytomegalovirus, herpes simplex, atypical mycobacteria, Kaposi's sarcoma

Radiology

In acute severe illness **a plain abdominal radiograph** is sufficient to diagnose the extent and severity of large bowel disease. Gas and the absence of residue occur in inflamed colon and allow the extent to be determined. If the colon cannot be visualized because there is no gas, air can be introduced via a rigid procto-sigmoidoscope and a further plain film obtained.

In an acute illness the extent of colonic inflammation can also be determined by a double contrast barium enema without bowel preparation ('**instant enema**') (page 17).

In fulminant colitis the colon may dilate ('**toxic megacolon**'). A diameter of greater than 6.5 cm is abnormal. The presence of **mucosal islands** indicates severe inflammation due to detached mucosa.

In long-standing ulcerative colitis the colon may become tubular and shortened due to the loss of haustrations.

A **barium follow-through** or **small bowel enema** examination allows the extent of small bowel Crohn's disease to be determined. The main features are:

> • Thickening of the valvulae conniventes
> • Oedema of the wall
> • Ulcers and fissuring
> • Lumenal narrowing and strictures
> • Prestenotic dilatation indicating a severe stricture
> • Fistulae to other structures or the skin

Rectal biopsy

A rectal biopsy can be obtained at the initial sigmoidoscopic examination. This should be taken from the posterior wall of the rectum below 10 cm, under direct vision, using small biopsy cup forceps.

Rectal and colonic biopsies should be examined for the nature of inflammation (ulcerative colitis versus Crohn's disease), collagenous colitis or microscopic inflammation if the macroscopic appearance is normal, and infection (Figures 5 and 6).

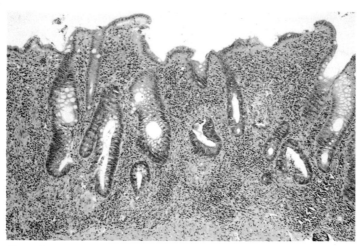

Figure 5
Ulcerative colitis histology showing distorted epithelial architecture with branched crypts, epithelial ulceration, crypt abscess and inflammatory infiltrate in lamina propria.

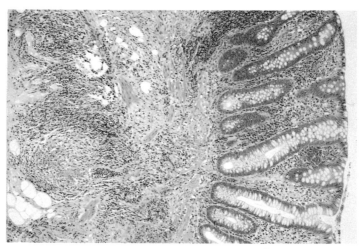

Figure 6
Crohn's disease histology showing preserved mucosal architecture, inflammatory infiltrate in the lamina propria and a deep granuloma.

Blood tests

Anaemia may be present in either condition, due to blood loss (iron deficiency), chronic inflammation (hypochromic or normocytic normochromic), or B_{12} malabsorption (macrocytic) in Crohn's disease. **Hypoalbuminaemia** suggests severe disease.

> The best markers of disease severity in Crohn's disease are elevation of the C-reactive protein and platelet count

Corticosteroids

Steroids are of proven efficacy in acute colitis and remain the standard by which other drugs are judged. Their introduction in the 1950s, together with appropriately timed surgery, drastically reduced the mortality of severe episodes of ulcerative colitis and Crohn's disease from about 50% to 1–2%. Steroids modify almost every part of the inflammatory response, including cell-mediated immunity and the production of most inflammatory mediators. Their biological effect lasts longer than their plasma half-life.

Oral steroids

The optimum initial dose of oral prednisolone for acute episodes of IBD is 40–60 mg per day in a single morning dose. Some patients who do not respond to 40 mg will respond to 60 mg per day.

Most patients tolerate short courses of oral steroids extremely well without side-effects. Occasional side-effects include:

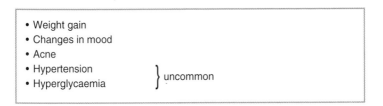

- Weight gain
- Changes in mood
- Acne
- Hypertension
- Hyperglycaemia } uncommon

These problems can be minimized by reducing the dose quickly as an acute episode is brought under control.

Long-term steroid use is associated with an increased risk of:

- Bone necrosis (e.g. femoral head)
- Osteoporosis (with increased risk of vertebral collapse and other fractures)
- Growth retardation in children

Steroids are not effective in maintaining remission and should not be used for prolonged periods.

New steroids

A recent therapeutic approach involves the use of steroids which are either poorly absorbed from the gastrointestinal tract and act directly on the mucosa, or are absorbed but rapidly metabolized on first pass through the mucosa or liver.

Budesonide

Budesonide is completely absorbed, has topical potency, and extensive first-pass metabolism. The systemic bioavailability after oral administration is about 10% in healthy volunteers, and about 15% after rectal administration. It is available in three forms:

- Entocort capsules designed to delay release of budesonide until the drug reaches the ileum, at which point there is a slow release throughout the ileocaecal region — for the treatment of ileocaecal Crohn's disease
- Budenofalk capsules— pH-modified release budesonide for Crohn's disease
- Entocort budesonide enema — for the treatment of distal ulcerative colitis

Budesonide results in significantly less adrenal suppression than oral prednisolone, in addition to a reduction in other steroid side-effects. In view of the concern about bone demineralization in patients with Crohn's disease, and the prospect of requiring repeated courses of steroids throughout these patients' lifetimes, an attempt should be made to minimize the loss of bone-mineral density when treating episodes of inflammation.

In addition, as treatment with budesonide results in lower systemic steroid levels than conventional oral steroid therapy the use of budesonide in place of oral prednisolone may also be considered when a patient has previously experienced the following on steroids:

- Mood changes or other CNS effects
- Hypertension
- Diabetes
- Cushingoid features
- Acne

Every attempt should be made to conserve bone density in patients who are known to have, or are at high risk of developing, osteoporosis. This includes patients who require frequent courses of steroids or women who are postmenopausal.

The recommended daily dose for the induction of remission in patients with mild to moderate Crohn's disease affecting the terminal ileum and/or ascending colon is 9 mg for up to 8 weeks. The dose should normally be tapered over the last 2–4 weeks of therapy. Budesonide is most effective when administered as a single morning dose, rather than in divided doses, possibly because higher mucosal drug levels are attained.

Other new steroids

Other topically active steroids, which have been mainly evaluated in enema form, include:

- Prednisolone sodium metasulphobenzoate – poorly absorbed and extensive first-pass metabolism
- Beclomethasone dipropionate – absorbed but rapidly metabolized by the liver
- Tixocortol pivalate – high first-pass metabolism by the liver; relatively low topical potency

Intravenous steroids

Severe episodes which are unresponsive to oral steroids may respond to intravenous treatment. The dose for intravenous treatment is methyl-prednisolone 20 mg three times per day.

Rectal steroid preparations

Rectal preparations act via a local effect on the mucosa.

Steroid enemas

- Prednisolone sodium metasulphobenzoate 20 mg (Predenema)
- Prednisolone-21-phosphate (or prednisolone sodium phosphate) 20 mg (Predsol)
- Budesonide 2 mg (Entocort enema)

Prednisolone metasulphobenzoate is absorbed less than prednisolone-21-phosphate. Budesonide enemas cause less adrenal suppression than prednisolone or hydrocortisone enemas. Enemas have good mucosal contact and are often more effective than foam — use them for disease extending as far proximal as the splenic flexure.

Steroid foam

- Prednisolone sodium metasulphobenzoate 20 mg (Predfoam)
- Hydrocortisone acetate 125 mg (Colifoam)

These two drugs are equivalent in potency. Foam is more easily retained than enema, especially if used during the day. They do not spread more proximally than the rectosigmoid.

Prednisolone suppository (5 mg)
This is useful for proctitis limited to the lowermost 10 cm of the rectum.

5-amino salicylic acid compounds

5-amino salicylic acid (5-ASA) compounds are mildly effective in acute episodes when given orally. Rectal preparations are as effective as steroids in acute episodes, and in some patients they are more effective. They are sometimes effective for episodes of proctitis that have not responded to steroid enemas. Some patients find them harder to retain than steroid enemas, but the ability to retain these enemas generally improves over a few days.

The great value of 5-ASA drugs is their ability to maintain remission in ulcerative colitis, and to a lesser extent in Crohn's disease. 5-ASA (also called mesalazine or mesalamine) acts locally on mucosa; it is readily absorbed from the small bowel, and must therefore be linked to another compound, or resin-coated, to be released at the site of inflammation. It acts at many points in the inflammatory process.

Sulphasalazine

Sulphasalazine is the longest established 5-ASA compound. It contains 5-ASA linked to sulphapyridine by an azo bond, which is split by bacteria in the terminal ileum and colon.

Its side-effects (headaches and nausea) are often dose-related and can sometimes be overcome by using an enteric-coated form. Sulphasalazine should not be used in patients with an allergy to sulphurs. Other side-effects include skin rashes and reversible male infertility due to oligospermia. Fifteen per cent of patients do not tolerate it.

More recent 5-ASA compounds

These do not contain a sulphur component. They are just as effective as sulphasalazine and are often better tolerated. Differences between the more recent 5-ASA compounds relate to different delivery mechanisms, resulting in some differences in the site of release and maximum concentration.

Mesalazine
This comes in two forms:

- Coated with the resin 'Eudragit-S' (Asacol) which dissolves at the pH (pH 7) found in the terminal ileum and colon
- Slow-release, ethylcellulose-coated microparticles (Pentasa) which are released throughout the small bowel and colon

Olsalazine (Dipentum)

Olsalazine consists of two 5-ASA molecules joined by an azo bond which is split by colonic bacteria. Because each molecule contains two 5-ASA components, the effective dose of 5-ASA delivered to the colon is higher than other similar drugs. Olsalazine can induce diarrhoea owing to a secretory effect in the small intestine, and should therefore be introduced slowly and taken with meals.

Balsalazide (Colazide)

This consists of a 5-ASA molecule bound to an inert carrier by an azo bond. 5-ASA is released in the colon in the same way as sulphasalazine (see page 37) but without the sulphur side-effects. Clinical trials have shown it to be at least as effective as other 5-ASA preparations, and with a low frequency of side-effects.

The 5-ASA drugs are rarely associated with **nephrotoxicity**; this is sometimes irreversible, thought to be idiosyncratic, and most commonly due to interstitial nephritis.

Azathioprine and 6-mercaptopurine

Azathioprine is metabolized to 6-mercaptopurine in vivo. This drug is valuable for patients who have frequent relapses despite taking a 5-ASA compound, as well as for patients with chronic active disease which flares up when steroids are reduced. It is of proven value in both ulcerative colitis and Crohn's disease.

The mode of action of azathioprine in IBD is uncertain. The drug does have an effect on lymphoid cell populations, and some of these changes are slow to occur, paralleling the long duration of treatment required to have a clinical effect.

The optimum dose of azathioprine is 2 mg/kg/day, and at least 4 months of therapy are required for the drug to have its maximum effect. In some patients up to 6 months of treatment is required for the drug to have an effect. Azathioprine can be started on its own, or as steroids are slowly tapered after an acute flare-up, or as steroids are slowly withdrawn in someone who has been taking them for a long time.

A minority of patients will not be maintained in remission and do not appear to benefit from the standard dose of 2 mg/kg/day. If their white cell count is maintained within the normal range, a proportion of these patients will benefit from an increase in dose to 2.5 or occasionally 3 mg/kg/day.

The clinical effect of azathioprine may be achieved more quickly if the drug is given initially as a large single loading infusion in a dose of 50 mg/kg over 2 days, to be followed by the usual oral dose. Caution is required, since some patients have an inherited low level of enzyme activity to metabolize the drug. Further data from clinical trials are awaited.

About 6% of patients cannot tolerate the drug because of nausea or vomiting, a flu-like syndrome, drug fever, or pancreatitis. To avoid leucopenia a blood count should be done every 2 weeks initially and thereafter monthly. Falls in the white cell count are reversible on stopping the drug.

When a patient has been well maintained in remission for 1 or 2 years on a standard dose of 2 mg/kg/day it may be possible to lower the dose and still maintain the patient in remission. Azathioprine maintains its efficacy for at least 4 or 5 years, and probably for longer. Attempts should be made to decrease the dose or stop using the drug after this time, although many patients will relapse on stopping the drug even after long-term therapy. Some of these patients will elect to go back on azathioprine to restore their well-being.

In renal transplant patients taking this drug there is a significant increase in malignancy. However, in IBD the dose used, the use of associated immunosuppressive drugs and the nature of immune system changes are different, and the risk of malignancy does not appear to be increased in patients with IBD. However, it is wise to suspend use of the drug after 3 or 4 years of therapy if possible.

Mycophenolate mofetil

Preliminary controlled studies suggest that mycophenolate mofetil is as effective as azathioprine in treating chronic active Crohn's disease. Mycophenolate mofetil may exert its effect faster than azathioprine, within 1 or 2 months. This drug should be considered for the patient who requires strong immunosuppression but is intolerant of azathioprine.

Side-effects include nausea and vomiting, and skin rashes. In the dose used for inflammatory bowel disease it is less clear whether there is the same degree of bone-marrow suppression as occurs with azathioprine; monitoring of the blood count is therefore advisable with a blood count every 2 weeks initially and thereafter monthly.

The drug is available in 250 mg and 500 mg preparations. The recommended dose at present in inflammatory bowel disease is 15 mg/kg/day, with a total dose of approximately 1500 mg per day. This dose is less than that used in transplant patients. It should be taken in two to three divided doses to decrease side-effects.

The drug has variable kinetics, and blood levels should therefore be monitored.

Methotrexate

Methotrexate is an anti-metabolite folic-acid inhibitor with both immunosuppressant and anti-inflammatory activity. The drug also has molecular homology to interleukin-1 and interferes with the inflammatory action of interleukin-2. Its greatest effect appears to be in patients with active disease who have had difficulty coming off steroids. Its side-effects are:

• Nausea	
• Diarrhoea	affecting about 10% of patients
• Stomatitis	
• Leucopenia	
• Elevation of liver function tests	
• Pneumonitis	
• Liver fibrosis (related to the cumulative dose)	

The dose which has been used in IBD is 25 mg intramuscularly once a week for short courses (12 weeks), followed by 7.5–15 mg orally per week. Up to 20% of patients will have side-effects which prevent its use. The beneficial effect of methotrexate is usually apparent within 2 to 4 weeks, allowing a quick assessment as to whether the drug is likely to help a particular patient.

Blood counts and liver function tests should initially be done every fortnight, and then monthly. The drug should be avoided when the risk of liver damage is increased — i.e. in patients with known liver disease, alcoholism, or obesity.

Cyclosporin

Cyclosporin is a potent inhibitor of cell-mediated immunity. It is very effective when administered intravenously for fulminant acute colitis, and will induce remission in at least 50% of patients who have failed to improve after treatment with intravenous steroids. It is as effective as intravenous steroids when used as a sole agent for severe disease. It has a valuable role in inducing remission for patients with fulminant colitis and for patients with chronic active severe disease.

The role of cyclosporin in Crohn's disease is less clear. For severe or fulminant disease it is sometimes useful when administered intravenously. For chronic active disease, controlled trials have given conflicting evidence, but the drug does appear helpful for some patients.

When used intravenously for severe disease the dose should be 2 mg/kg/day. Higher doses give an increased incidence of side effects. The whole blood level should be monitored, aiming for a trough level of 100–200 ng/ml.

Used orally, drug absorption is unpredictable, so monitoring of blood levels, renal function, and blood pressure is essential. Grapefruit juice modifies the metabolism of cyclosporin by the cytochrome P450 system, and should be avoided.

Leukotriene inhibitors

Steroids, chloroquine and lignocaine block the release of arachidonic acid from the membrane phospholipid. Inhibition of the enzyme 5-lipoxygenase may also reduce levels of LBT4.

Alternative substrates to arachidonic acid can result in the biosynthesis of alternative weaker inflammatory mediators such as LBT5. However, there is still substantial production of LBT4.

Double-blind studies of **fish oil** or **eicosapentaenoic acid** have produced moderate results in maintaining remission in both ulcerative colitis and Crohn's disease.

Selective **inhibition of 5-lipoxygenase** may reduce LBT4 production by 90% or more.

Cytokine modulators

Interleukin-1 may be modified by the use of IL-1 converting enzyme inhibition, or by supplementation of IL-1 receptor antagonist or soluble IL-1 receptors.

Interleukin-2 receptor monoclonal antibodies or chimeric IL-2 toxins may have a role in suppressing inflammation.

Interleukin-10 plays an important part in repairing the damage from inflammation. It is currently being evaluated in Crohn's disease. Early studies have shown a significant therapeutic effect in patients resistant to standard therapies.

Alpha interferon has been used in inflammatory bowel disease with mixed results. A high incidence of severe side-effects has limited its use.

Antibodies directed against **tumour necrosis factor (TNF)**, given in a single dose, appear to have a dramatic and sustained effect in inducing remission in patients with resistant active Crohn's disease. A small proportion of patients will develop endogenous antibodies against these exogenously administered antibodies, but the significance of this is unknown. Until there is greater experience these drugs should be reserved for patients resistant to standard medications.

Tumour necrosis factor alpha (TNF-alpha) antibody treatment has been shown to induce remission in two thirds of patients with Crohn's disease resistant to standard therapies. This treatment has also maintained remission in two thirds of initially responsive patients over a 12-month period, when given as a single infusion every 8 weeks. The incidence of developing endogenous antibodies to the drug is low, and is not clinically significant. The long-term effects and benefits remain to be determined.

Lymphocyte modifiers

Administered **CD4 antibodies** may have a prolonged and marked effect on disease activity, but does lead to prolonged depletion of CD4 cells.

Plasmapheresis to remove selective lymphocyte populations is unlikely to have a major role due to the invasiveness, expense and dubious benefit of the treatment.

Miscellaneous drugs used in IBD

Topical short chain fatty acids in enema form are effective in treating diversion colitis, when the distal large bowel has been defunctioned. They are not useful in other forms of inflammation.

Antituberculous therapy is used in the belief that Crohn's disease may be due to an atypical mycobacterium, but has not produced sustained remissions in Crohn's disease, and has no established role in this condition.

Ciprofloxacin may be helpful in some patients with ulcerative colitis or perianal Crohn's disease.

Hydroxychloroquine is no better than placebo in treating patients with ulcerative colitis, despite 4-aminoquinolones affecting T-cell function.

Topical lignocaine appears to modify inflammation in patients with colitis, possibly by modifying the neural component of inflammation or by affecting the release of ecosanoids. May be useful in patients with distal colitis.

Bismuth subsalicylate enemas may be as effective as steroid and 5-ASA enemas, as seen in a small number of controlled studies. May therefore have a useful role in patients who have not responded to first-line treatments.

Hyperbaric oxygen may be useful for patients with resistant perineal Crohn's disease, although all the studies of its use have been uncontrolled.

Heparin may have a specific immunomodulatory effect — currently being evaluated for acute use. Osteoporosis precludes long-term use. Other coagulation pathway factors, such as factor XIII, are also being evaluated.

Reactive oxygen metabolites may be important in the genesis of tissue injury. Compounds that block the release or effects of these metabolites are being tested.

Drug therapy

Ulcerative colitis (Figure 7)

Acute episodes

For very mild flare-ups an increase in the dose of oral 5-ASA drugs may be helpful. Otherwise, steroids form the first-line treatment for acute disease.

Proctitis (inflammation confined to the lower 10 cm of the rectum)
Suppositories are usually effective:

> - Start with prednisolone (5 mg)
> - If ineffective use mesalazine (250 mg or 500 mg)

Severe episodes
These may require a short course of oral prednisolone.

Rectosigmoid or left colonic inflammation
Enemas are usually effective when used each night. They should extend as far proximally as the descending colon or splenic flexure. If the whole 100 ml cannot be retained then use

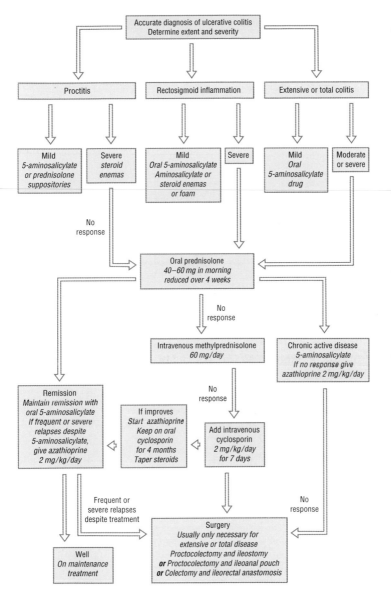

Figure 7
Treatment pathways for patients with ulcerative colitis.

a smaller volume initially, or a foam. For more severe episodes, prednisolone foam can be added during the day, after the patient has completed going to the toilet.

- Start with prednisolone 20 mg enema
- If not tolerated use prednisolone or hydrocortisone foam
- Use mesalazine enema or foam if no response to steroid

Steroid enemas are usually effective and reassure the patient that their disease can be relatively easily controlled. However, mesalazine enemas are equally effective and can be tried in subsequent episodes, although some patients find them more difficult to retain. Occasionally they are very effective in patients who have not responded to steroid enemas.

Patients who cannot tolerate a rectal 5-aminosalicylate preparation and who have not responded to one of the standard fixed-dose steroid enemas can make up a steroid enema to an increased concentration. Six or more soluble 5mg prednisolone-21-phosphate tablets can be dissolved in 100 ml (or less initially if 100 ml not tolerated) warm tapwater in a 100 ml syringe with a soft rubber tubing nozzle (Figure 8). Once the condition is under control the dose can be decreased. Many patients like the convenience of these self-administered steroid enemas when travelling, as they need only to carry a syringe and a packet of tablets.

Severe proctitis or distal colitis
This is characterized by:

- High bowel frequency (6–8 per day or more)
- Rectal bleeding
- Severe inflammation on sigmoidoscopy
- More marked systemic symptoms

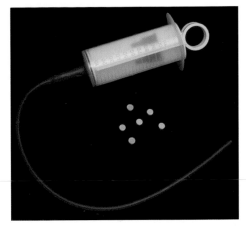

Figure 8
100 ml irrigating syringe that can be used to make up a steroid enema. Soluble prednisolone sodium phosphate (Prednesol) tablets are dissolved in warm tapwater. If the patient does not respond to 20 mg drug, the dose can be increased to 30 mg. If the patient cannot tolerate 100 ml solution, then smaller volumes such as 50 ml can be used initially.

Severe episodes usually require oral steroids, as enemas are not retained. Rarely, intravenous steroids are required: change to oral steroids as patient responds, and when tapering is nearly complete consider reintroducing enemas or foam to maintain control as the dose is reduced.

Extensive or total colitis

Very mild episodes may respond to a substantial dose of a 5-ASA drug, such as 6 or more tablets per day. However, most acute episodes require oral prednisolone in a dose of 40–60 mg per day.

Severe episodes, characterized by a high bowel frequency, fever, tachycardia, or other significant systemic symptoms, require hospital admission and treatment with intravenous steroids. There is no added benefit from routine use of antibiotics or food restriction.

For severe episodes that fail to respond to intravenous steroids, the addition of intravenous cyclosporin (2–5 mg/kg/day) is effective in more than half of all patients. Intravenous cyclosporin without steroids may also be effective here. The lower dose of 2 mg/kg/day appears to be as effective as higher doses, and is associated with far fewer side-effects. It should be administered intravenously for 7–10 days. The effect is rapid and clinical response is usually apparent within 3–5 days. Patients who fail therapy with intravenous cyclosporin for fulminant disease require surgical treatment.

After successful intravenous therapy oral cyclosporin should be continued for 3–4 months, whilst waiting for azathioprine to take effect. Oral cyclosporin (Neoral) should be given initially in a dose of 4–5 mg/kg/day (divided into twice daily doses) and then adjusted so that the trough morning blood level is between 100 and 200 ng/ml. Azathioprine should be started while the patient is still in hospital.

Assessing the response to treatment

The success of treatment of individual episodes is based on:

- Relief of symptoms, especially bowel frequency, bleeding and a sense of well-being
- Improvement in the sigmoidoscopic appearance

Eighty per cent of acute episodes, regardless of the extent of disease, improve substantially with treatment in 2 weeks. The dose of medication should then be tapered over the subsequent 3 or 4 weeks, providing that the condition continues to improve. In many patients, worsening of an episode occurs as the drug dose or frequency is reduced; the dose should then be temporarily increased until symptoms improve, and then the dose should be decreased more slowly.

Maintaining remission

When relapses occur more than once a year an oral 5-ASA drug should be taken long term.

5-ASA drugs can reduce the relapse rate in ulcerative colitis from 70% to 20% in one year, and this efficacy is maintained long term. The prevention of recurrence is proportional to the dose.

Commonly used doses to prevent relapse are:

- Sulphasalazine (Salazopyrin) 1 g twice a day
- Olsalazine (Dipentum) 0.5–1 g twice a day (achieves high colonic concentrations)
- Mesalazine (Asacol) 800 mg (two tablets) two to three times a day
- Slow-release mesalazine (Pentasa) 500 mg three times a day

If a patient still relapses frequently or has chronic active disease despite adequate doses of a 5-ASA drug, then azathioprine therapy can be started

Crohn's disease

Acute episodes
Left-sided or total colitis

The drug management of acute colonic Crohn's disease is identical to that in ulcerative colitis (see above), with the exception that in severe Crohn's disease the use of intravenous cyclosporin in patients who would otherwise require colectomy is unproven, although anecdotal evidence suggests that it may be useful.

Crohn's proctitis

Simple Crohn's proctitis is treated in the same way as ulcerative proctitis. However, Crohn's proctitis is more liable to stricture formation, especially if there is marked anal involvement.

Perianal disease

Abscesses need to be treated by surgical drainage. For **anal fissure** and **chronic anal suppuration**, try steroid ointment applied intra-anally and perianally and prednisolone suppositories.

Chronic fistulae in the absence of abscess formation should initially be treated with metronidazole 400 mg twice to three times a day. This should not be used for longer than 4–8 weeks due to the risk of peripheral neuropathy. **Severe cases** may require a course of oral steroids. If fistulae are persistent and severe, introduce maintenance azathioprine therapy. For **acute severe disease** use cyclosporin 2–5 mg/kg/day intravenously.

Localized terminal ileal disease

This is the most common isolated form of Crohn's disease. It may respond to intermittent courses of oral budesonide or prednisolone. Budesonide gives less adrenal suppression and less bone demineralization, and causes fewer steroid side-effects than prednisolone. Budesonide should be started at 9 mg daily for up to 8 weeks; alternatively prednisolone should be started in a dose of 40–60 mg per day.

If a patient is unresponsive to short courses of steroid therapy, or has frequent relapses despite an oral 5-ASA and azathioprine, they may require surgery. This group of patients has the best outcome with surgical resection.

Extensive small bowel disease

This can be the most difficult to treat. Acute episodes should be treated with short courses of steroids. Slow-release mesalazine 4 g daily can be used for mild acute disease. For recurrent disease or chronic active disease use azathioprine.

If the condition is unresponsive to drugs try liquid diet and food exclusion (see page 57) for 4–6 weeks. Start slow-release mesalazine or azathioprine as the patient improves, to maintain remission.

Mouth ulcers

These usually respond to hydrocortisone lozenges. If more troublesome, combine steroid lozenges with 2–3 times daily antiseptic mouth wash, as ulcers tend to be the result of a combination of oral Crohn's disease and bacterial infection. Occasionally, if very severe, mouth ulcers may require treatment with oral steroids. If very severe and recurrent, azathioprine treatment may be required.

Post-resection diarrhoea

After ileal and proximal colon resection many patients have 3–4 loose bowel actions per day. If this is troublesome, some patients respond to cholestyramine for bile salt overflow, or loperamide.

Maintaining remission

Mesalazine in slow-release or locally releasing (if colonic disease) formulation, will increase the remission rate. Doses of at least 2 g daily are required.

For patients who relapse despite high dose 5-ASA, or who have more severe chronic active disease, use azathioprine 2 mg/kg/day.

Pouchitis (Figure 9)

Initial treatment should be metronidazole 400–800 mg twice daily for 10 days. Clinical improvement usually occurs within 48 hours.

Patients who have frequent relapses can be given low dose metronidazole, such as 200 mg each second day, but many patients experience nausea with this drug, and irreversible peripheral neuropathy is a concern with long-term use.

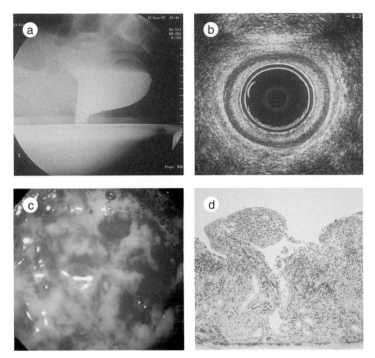

Figure 9

A woman aged 30 had an ileoanal pouch for 2 years after previous ulcerative colitis. She had 10 loose bowel actions during the day and 3 episodes of incontinence each night. She has had two vaginal deliveries in the past.

(a) Lateral pouchogram shows a good sized pouch; thus a small reservoir capacity was not the cause for her symptoms.

(b) Anal endosonography. This scan is a horizontal section through the mid anal canal. The central area is the endosonographic probe. Surrounding this is the white ring of anal mucosa. Lateral to this is the dark ring of the internal anal sphincter smooth muscle. Lateral to this is the white heterogeneous appearance of the external anal sphincter. Both sphincter muscles are circumferentially intact, excluding structural damage from childbirth or from the bowel surgery as the cause of her incontinence.

(c) Endoscopic examination shows severe pouchitis with macroscopic epithelial ulceration.

(d) Haematoxylin and eosin stained section of pouch mucosal biopsy, showing an erosion of the pouch ileal epithelium and mucosal inflammatory cell infiltrate.

If metronidazole is unsuccessful, topical treatments (as used in distal ulcerative colitis) are usually successful. These include steroid or 5-ASA suppositories, foam, or enemas. Rarely, oral 5-ASA drugs or steroids are required. For patients with recurrent or severe disease azathioprine may be required.

Preliminary studies suggest that eliminating the bowel flora using wide-spectrum antibiotics, and replacing it with probiotic formulations of bacteria and yeasts, may maintain patients with resistant pouchitis in remission. Further studies are awaited to confirm this.

Collagenous colitis/microscopic (lymphocytic) colitis and microscopic polymorphonuclear inflammation

Most patients respond to an oral 5-ASA drug. Rarely, a short course of oral steroids is required.

Microscopic polymorph inflammation will often declare itself as overt macroscopic ulcerative colitis or Crohn's disease, sometimes only after a period of years.

Diet and nutritional therapy

Crohn's disease

Children and adolescents

> Inadequate nutrition is the major cause of impaired growth
> in children and adolescents with Crohn's disease

In children and adolescents, height and weight should be
recorded regularly and plotted on a commercially available
graph of normal values. Impaired growth velocity requires nutritional therapy. This may form the main treatment, or may be
used in combination with drugs or surgery.

Steroid therapy is less important than inadequate nutrition in
impairing growth, and can be used in short courses.

Liquid diet supplementation

Nutritional supplementation, orally or via nocturnal nasogastric
feeding, can have a dramatic effect on growth and allow catch-
ing-up. Such treatment should be given before the opportunity
is lost due to epiphyseal fusion.

An effective means of supplementing nutrient consumption is to get the child, adolescent, or adult patient to pass a fine-bore nasogastric tube each evening. Some 1000–1500 ml (supplying up to 1500 ml Kcal) of liquid diet can then be infused overnight, regulated with a pump.

There is also good evidence that improving nutritional status alone can lessen Crohn's disease activity, and that dietary modification can improve symptoms and reduce inflammation.

Liquid diet enteral feeding as food replacement

Liquid diets, when taken as the only enteral source of nutrition, improve Crohn's disease activity.

Commercially available liquid diets vary in their protein, carbohydrate, and fat content. Proteins may consist of a limited number of simple proteins (polymeric diets), hydrolysed proteins, or aminoacids (elemental diets). Polymeric diets (whole proteins, polysaccharides, and fat) appear to be as good as elemental diets (aminoacids, glucose, and little fat, with minerals and vitamins), and are more palatable. Elemental diets usually need to be given by nasogastric tube, but polymeric diets are often tolerated well orally.

Liquid diets with a low fat content may have a superior effect on inflammation, possibly because they provide less substrate for the inflammatory process.

If patients can tolerate a purified liquid diet (orally or via nasogastric feeding) many can achieve induction of remission, although the response rate of 75% is slightly less than that achieved by steroids.

For simplicity, steroids are usually the first-line approach, but dietary therapy may be helpful in children with growth problems or patients resistant to steroid treatment. A polymeric diet should be tried first.

When a liquid diet is the sole nutritional source, this is usually undertaken for 4–8 weeks. Approximately 75% of patients will achieve remission. In children approximately half of these will relapse within 6 months and 60% will relapse within 12 months. This relapse rate can be reduced if nasogastric feeding is continued after resumption of an otherwise normal diet.

Percutaneous gastrostomy supplementation or feeding

When oral or nasogastric feeding is not tolerated and nutritional support is required, a percutaneous endoscopic gastrostomy tube can be inserted. The complication rate and safety are the same in Crohn's disease as in other conditions, providing there is no sepsis present at the time of insertion. There is no increased rate of gastrocutaneous fistulae after tube removal.

Liquid feeding via a percutaneous gastrostomy can be used either to supply a liquid diet as the sole source of dietary intake, or to supplement normal oral intake. In addition to inducing remission when used alone, a continued liquid diet supplementation when a normal diet is resumed allows for a longer remission.

Intravenous nutrition with bowel rest

Complete bowel rest with cessation of oral intake replaced by intravenous feeding will allow improvement in most patients with severe disease, but is associated with a significant complication rate, especially sepsis. A clinical remission of at least 1 year occurs in 60% of patients. Intravenous feeding alone has no clear advantage over allowing patients also to take an enteral liquid diet, and enteral diets are now the preferred form of therapy.

Food

Although patients with Crohn's disease eat more sugar than normal, reducing this sugar intake does not produce clinical benefit.

Food sensitivities vary between patients with Crohn's disease, but commonly incriminated foods include:

- Nuts
- Raw fruits
- Green vegetables
- Tomatoes
- Alcohol
- Wheat products
- Dairy products

Exclusion diets are of unproven value in inducing or maintaining remission.

Ulcerative colitis

There are no proven dietary therapies for ulcerative colitis, nor are there any proven dietary components that consistently aggravate the disease. However, some patients find avoiding wheat products or dairy products helpful.

Ulcerative colitis

There are three surgical options:

- Proctocolectomy and ileostomy
- Colectomy with ileorectal anastomosis
- Restorative proctocolectomy with ileoanal reservoir ('pouch')

Proctocolectomy and ileostomy

This option has several advantages. It:

- Is the simplest operation
- Involves only one operation
- Incurs the lowest morbidity and mortality

For patients who are happy to have a stoma this is a good operation. Even with an ileostomy, however, there is morbidity, with a readmission rate of 45% over 10 years. The complications of a stoma are listed in Table 3.

Complication	Frequency
Skin problems	34%
Intestinal obstruction	23%
Retraction	17%
Parastomal herniation	16%

Table 3
Long-term complications of an ileostomy.

Colectomy with ileorectal anastomosis

Colostomy with ileorectal anastomosis can be useful for the older patient who needs a colectomy, has relative rectal sparing, and who could not cope with a stoma. It is *not* suitable for:

- Young patients with total colitis, because of the 15% lifetime cancer risk in the rectum. It can be used in these patients as an interim measure with a view to creating a pouch later
- Patients with marked rectal inflammation, as they will continue to experience urgency, diarrhoea, and bleeding

Restorative proctocolectomy with ileoanal reservoir ('pouch')

This procedure allows patients to maintain continence. It is a more complex operation, with a high perioperative morbidity. Sepsis around the anastomosis is a common perioperative problem, occurring in about 30% of patients, although it usually resolves. A covering stoma is sometimes required, with ileostomy closure 2–3 months later. This may result in a total of two or three operations (proctocolectomy, pouch formation, ileostomy closure). If the operation fails then some small intestine may be lost.

The pouch is created using the distal small intestine. It is sewn or stapled together to form a reservoir which can then be anastomosed to the anal canal. The most common designs are a 'J' or a 'W' pouch, the latter being slightly larger (Figure 10).

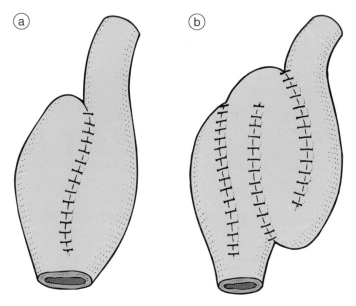

Figure 10
(a) The 'J' pouch.
(b) The 'W' pouch. The former has slightly less capacity than the latter, but their function is similar.

It is now 20 years since the first pouch operations, and the long-term outcome is better known. Approximately 15% of patients will need to have the pouch removed, due to sepsis, fistulae, other technical problems, incontinence, or pouchitis. Chronic active intractable pouchitis occurs in about 5% of patients.

Crohn's disease

Surgery in Crohn's disease is reserved for complications of the disease, or for severe disease of limited anatomical extent which is unresponsive to conservative treatment.

Indications for surgery include:

- Abscess that cannot be treated by percutaneous drainage
- Obstruction that is unrelieved by drug therapy
- Enterocutaneous fistula
- A limited segment of diseased intestine causing severe symptoms despite maximum medical therapy
- Perianal infection requiring drainage

Terminal ileal resection

Young adults with disease limited to 10–20 cm of terminal ileum often do well with a limited resection that includes the caecum and appendix. Although most patients remain asymptomatic for some years after this procedure, endoscopic studies have shown that anastomotic disease recurrence occurs in at least 80% of patients within 6 months.

Strictureplasty

Extensive resections of diseased intestine can result in a short intestine. Mini-resection or strictureplasty should therefore be done where possible. Strictureplasty involves making a longitudinal incision along a small intestinal stricture and resuturing transversely. Strictureplasty relieves obstruction and in many cases the disease regresses at the operative site.

Enterocutaneous fistula

Nutritional, metabolic, and fluid support are the mainstays of treating fistulae. Surgery is usually required to resect diseased intestine. Postoperative fistulae often resolve with bowel rest and parenteral nutrition.

Colonic disease

For severe colonic disease and rectal sparing a **colectomy with ileorectal anastomosis** is possible, but the recurrence rate is double that of a terminal ileostomy.

Severe perianal or colonic disease sometimes requires a diverting ileostomy, but in the long term only a quarter of patients treated in this way have their intestinal continuity restored.

Prevention of postoperative recurrence

Long-term 5-aminosalicylates and azathioprine, and a 3-month postoperative course of metronidazole all reduce the post-operative recurrence rate after curative resection of macro-scopically diseased bowel.

A practical approach is to give 5-aminosalicylates to all patients, especially after resections where all macroscopically affected tissue is thought to have been removed. The dose should be at least 2 g daily of a preparation which releases at the appropriate site. This preparation should be slow-release for most patients, or a pH coated or azo bond preparation for those with colonic disease.

For patients who have already had one postoperative recurrence, or who have residual inflammation after resection, long-term therapy with azathioprine should be considered.

Endoscopic balloon dilatation

Patients with anastomotic recurrence and stricturing, or with stricturing owing to a short segment of active inflammation, may be amenable to endoscopic balloon dilatation (Figure 11). For many patients this will avoid the need for surgical treatment.

The stricture should be radiologically imaged first, to ensure:

- It is accessible endoscopically
- It Is short
- There is widely patent intestine proximal to the stricture
- The intestine is not angulated, so that a balloon may be passed safely across the stricture

Given these conditions the stricture should be dilated progressively using fixed diameter balloons that pass down the biopsy channel. A 10 mm diameter balloon should be used first, eventually reaching a maximum diameter of 18 mm if safe.

Long-term studies have shown that such dilatations can be performed safely in the small and large intestine, and remain patent for several years.

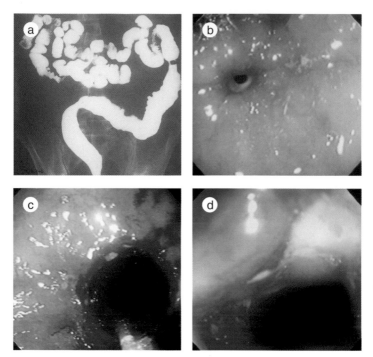

Figure 11
(a) Small bowel to left colon anastomotic stricture in a 43-year-old man with three previous operations for Crohn's disease and a relatively short small intestine. There is slight proximal dilatation, suggesting that this is of functional significance. The stricture is short, accessible, and suitable for dilating.
(b) Endoscopic view of the same stricture with a pin hole opening.
(c) Balloon dilated across the stricture.
(d) After dilatation the lumen is patent.

Fertility

Most patients with IBD have a normal ability to conceive and carry a pregnancy. Patients with Crohn's disease who have had extensive pelvic sepsis may have a reduced ability to conceive and a high risk of ectopic pregnancy.

Patients with diarrhoea should not rely solely on an oral contraceptive.

Patients on a 5-ASA drug to maintain remission should continue the drug when trying to conceive or when pregnant.

For patients on azathioprine advice needs to be tailored to the clinical situation and the patient allowed to make an informed choice. For patients who have had previous severe disease controlled with azathioprine, it may be reasonable to continue the drug during pregnancy. In others with mild disease it may be possible to substitute a 5-aminosalicylate preparation for azathioprine at the time of conception and pregnancy. Teratogenic effects from azathioprine have not been reported in patients treated for inflammatory bowel disease.

Pregnancy and lactation

Pregnancy does not adversely affect disease activity. Rarely, the disease may start in pregnancy or flare up soon after delivery.

Treatment of acute episodes is the same as for non-pregnant patients. Despite fears about the use of oral steroids during the first trimester, it is likely that an acute flare-up of inflammatory bowel disease is more threatening to the pregnancy than any theoretical risk from the drugs used. Use of systemic steroids in the first trimester has been associated with the development of cleft lip and palate.

5-ASA drugs are excreted in breast milk, but not in high concentration, and may be continued during lactation.

Children

The same treatment principles apply to children as to adults with ulcerative colitis. Immunosuppressive therapy is not contraindicated, but is more controversial because the child will have a longer projected duration of illness. This factor, together with impaired growth, occasionally lowers the threshold for consideration of surgery.

Inadequate nutrition is the most likely cause of impaired growth in children, especially in Crohn's disease (see page 56).

Faecal urgency and incontinence

For many patients the most distressing symptom and greatest social inconvenience of IBD is faecal urgency. This symptom occurs in patients with disease of any extent.

Urgency is most commonly seen when there is active disease, and the disease must be assessed and treated. Anti-diarrhoeal drugs should not be taken in the presence of acute inflammation. In addition to bowel inflammation, contributing causes include obstetric sphincter damage in women and sphincter damage in patients who have had anal disease.

Urgency occasionally persists when there is low grade chronic active disease or when the patient is in remission. Providing that marked inflammation has been excluded, this symptom can sometimes be significantly relieved by the judicious use of a small morning dose of loperamide (2–4 mg) or codeine phosphate (15 or 30 mg). The risk of addiction is negligible.

Faecal urgency and incontinence may not always be caused by the inflammatory bowel disease, especially if still present when the disease is quiescent. Other causes, such as sphincter damage related to childbirth, anal surgery, and previous inflammation and sepsis, should be considered and excluded.

Short bowel syndrome

Intestinal resections for Crohn's disease (see page 63) can result in an inadequate length of intestine to maintain adequate fluid or nutritional balance. Even one resection can result in a short bowel if the small intestine is at the short end of the spectrum prior to resection. Resection for Crohn's disease is the commonest cause of short bowel syndrome.

Patients with an end jejunostomy or ileostomy will usually require:

- *Electrolyte supplementation* – if stoma output exceeds **1 litre per day** (usually a small intestinal length of less than 150 cm)

- *Intravenous (or occasionally nocturnal nasogastric) fluid supplementation* – if stoma output exceeds **1500 ml per day** (usually a small intestinal length of less than 120 cm)
- *Intravenous nutritional support* – if stoma output exceeds **2 litres per day**. This output reflects inadequate gut length (usually less than 100 cm small intestine) to absorb adequate fluid and nutrients. If the short small intestine is anastomosed to retained colon, the need for parenteral nutrition can be avoided if the patient has more than 50 cm undiseased small intestine

Replacing high stomal losses

Stomal losses are high in sodium content (isosmolar – 135 mmol/litre). Oral fluids should therefore be as high as possible in salt content; standard electrolyte replacements are inadequate because they contain the same sodium concentration as stool (30 mmol/litre).

The highest palatable concentration in a made-up electrolyte mix is 90 mmol/litre. Patients requiring this can be given a set of spoons to make up a 1 litre solution each morning containing 90 mmol/litre sodium (3.5 g NaCl), 20 g glucose and 2.5 g sodium bicarbonate.

Other requirements in patients on electrolyte supplementation

Patients requiring electrolyte mix often develop **hypomagnesaemia**. This can be replaced with magnesium oxide, although this sometimes aggravates stomal output.

Vitamin B_{12} needs to be replaced with 2-monthly injections in patients with terminal ileal resection.

Bone disease

Decreased bone density and osteoporosis

Patients with inflammatory bowel disease are at increased risk of bone demineralization and fractures. At first presentation, patients with Crohn's disease already have decreased bone density compared to age and sex matched healthy individuals. This is thought to relate mainly to the effect of disease activity on bone resorption, possibly via an effect of circulating proinflammatory cytokines on osteoclast activity. Genetic factors and hormone levels are also likely to be important. Patients with ulcerative colitis have normal bone density at first presentation.

Bone density is most commonly measured using dual energy X-ray absorptiometry (DEXA), usually in the lumbar spine, femoral head, and wrist. This technique has a high precision and a low radiation dose. Values are compared with a healthy young adult population (T score). A reasonable agreed definition for osteopenia is a T score of more than 1 standard deviation (SD) but less than 2.5 SD below the normal mean value for young adults of the same sex, with osteoporosis defined as more than 2.5 SD below the mean.

Factors which may contribute to bone demineralization in inflammatory bowel disease include:

- A direct effect of the inflammatory process on bone osteoclast activity
- Treatment with steroids
- Impaired vitamin D and calcium absorption. Impaired absorption is not the main factor in most patients, although in some ethnic groups it may be important
- Allelic variants of a number of genes such as the vitamin D receptor, oestrogen receptor, type 1 collagen, and TGF-beta
- Sex hormone deficiency
- Smoking, especially in women
- Malnutrition

In addition to the assessment of bone mineral density, an initial assessment should involve exclusion of osteomalacia, usually by measurement of serum calcium, vitamin D, and alkaline phosphatase.

Treatment with agents proven to increase bone density and decrease fracture rates should be seriously considered in patients who have inflammatory bowel disease and:

- Have a history of fractures
- Are postmenopausal, and receive more than one short course of steroids each year
- Receive frequent courses of steroids
- Have proven osteopenia or osteoporosis (T score below -1), even in the absence of previous fractures or further steroid treatment

If a decision has been made to treat bone demineralization, then the treatment used should depend on the patient's specific characteristics:

- If measured bone density is low, vitamin D, serum calcium, and alkaline phosphatase levels should be measured. Patients with malabsorption of vitamin D or calcium should be treated with supplemental calcium (calcium carbonate 1000 mg daily) and either vitamin D (250 IU daily) or calcitriol
- If vitamin D levels and serum calcium are normal, then consider hormone replacement therapy for postmenopausal women or premenopausal women with amenorrhoea
- If vitamin D levels and serum calcium are normal, then consider bisphosphonates in men and premenopausal women. This can be given as etidronate 400 mg daily for 2 weeks, followed by calcium 500 mg daily for 10 weeks, with four such cycles over a year. This sequential combination of etidronate and calcium is available prepackaged

Patients with decreased bone density should have bone density measurements at 1 or 2 year intervals.

The two main pharmaceutical interventions available at present, hormone replacement therapy and the bisphosphonates, both halve the fracture risk within the first 1–3 years of use.

Prevention

When systemic steroids are prescribed, the duration of treatment should be as short as is clinically practicable. If the disease distribution allows it, topically active steroids such as budesonide, with a lower systemic effect than prednisolone, should be used.

Even with enema treatment, the use of topically active steroids or 5-aminosalicylates should be considered.

Osteomalacia

This should always be excluded prior to the start of treatment of low bone mineral density.

A small number of patients will have osteomalacia. This may be due to low vitamin D levels, as seen in some ethnic groups. Alternatively, it can occur due to impaired calcium absorption, often related to extensive small bowel disease or a short small intestine. This requires specific treatment with calcium and vitamin D. Occasionally this needs to be given parenterally, especially in patients with a short gut syndrome.

Prognosis

Ulcerative colitis

Prior to the 1950s, one third of patients with a severe episode (initial or relapse) died. Improved management, parenteral therapy, fluid and electrolyte replacement, the timely use of surgery and the introduction of steroids have led to a reduction of mortality to negligible levels.

Twenty per cent of patients will have only one episode of inflammation, although a proportion of these episodes will have been undiagnosed infection and not ulcerative colitis.

Most patients have an intermittent relapsing course, although 20% will have chronic active disease. The chance of having chronic active disease, or even intermittent attacks, decreases with the time from onset.

Risk of progression of anatomical extent

The extent of disease at presentation is shown in Table 4. In 70% of patients with left-sided disease and in 34% of patients with inflammation of the rectum and sigmoid, disease will extend to involve most of the colon.

Extent	Frequency
Proctitis	33%
Rectosigmoid	35%
Left-sided disease	3%
Disease from the hepatic flexure	12%
Total colitis	16%

Table 4
Extent of disease at presentation.

Risk of colectomy

In patients with pancolitis:

- Risk of colectomy is 9% in the year of diagnosis
- Risk of colectomy is 3% per year in each of the following 4 years
- Risk of colectomy is 1% per year after that
- The cumulative colectomy rate after 15 years is 30%

Risk of cancer

The lifetime risk of colorectal cancer in the general population in Britain is 1 in 30, with an approximate risk of dying from colorectal cancer of 1 in 50. The lifetime risk for patients with ulcerative colitis is increased, depending on the nature of the disease (Table 5).

Increased risk vs general population	
All UC patients	x8
Total colitis	x19
Left-sided disease	x4
Distal disease	x1.5

Table 5
Increased risk of colorectal cancer in patients with ulcerative colitis.

The risk of colon cancer is greatest in ulcerative colitis in patients with:

- Disease for more than 8 years
- Disease extending from proximal to the splenic flexure

It is not known whether the number and severity of inflammatory episodes of colitis influence the risk of cancer, although one population-based study has suggested that tight control with 5-ASA drugs and a low threshold for colectomy reduce the cancer risk to that of the general population.

Other factors thought to be associated with an increased risk of cancer include:

- The presence of sclerosing cholangitis
- The presence of a dysplasia associated lesion or mass (DALM)
- A family history of colorectal cancer in a close relative, especially at a young age
- The presence of large bowel adenoma(s)

Surveillance

Surveillance programmes appear to be effective in preventing cancer in some patients by detecting premalignant high grade dysplasia, and by detecting cancer more often at an early stage when present. Five-year survival is increased in patients in whom cancer is detected in a surveillance programme, compared with those who develop cancer outside such a programme.

Until now surveillance programmes have utilized colonoscopically-obtained biopsies showing the histological presence of dysplasia as a marker for the likely development or presence of malignancy (Figure 12).

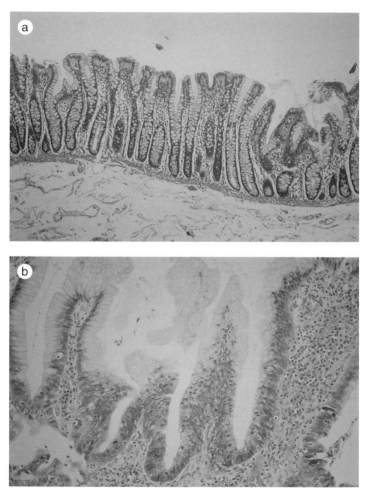

Figure 12
(a) Haematoxylin and eosin section of normal colonic mucosa
(b) High grade dysplasia in a patient with long-standing ulcerative colitis. Gross
abnormalities of intracellular and epithelial architecture.

High grade, and possibly definite low grade dysplasia, appear to be important predictors of the transformation to malignancy, or the presence of coexistent malignancy. However, dysplasia is not an infallible marker as it is absent in 25% of patients who have colorectal cancer.

Markers of malignant potential that are likely to be useful in the future include:

- Presence of DNA aneuploidy (measured by flow cytometry)
- p53 heterozygosity
- Presence of other tumour markers

Current recommendations for cancer surveillance include:

- **Establishing the anatomical extent** of inflammation after 8 years of inflammation, preferably by colonoscopy if no upper limit can be seen sigmoidoscopically. This should be done when mild (not severe or absent) inflammation is present
- **Colonoscopy done each year** in patients with disease extending proximal to the splenic flexure
- **Biopsies** taken from at least every 10 cm as well as any suspicious areas

Regular colonoscopy may also be indicated for patients with left-sided or distal disease who also have other coexisting risk factors such as a strong family history of colon cancer, the presence of sclerosing cholangitis, or the presence of adenomatous polyps.

Colectomy is advisable if definite high grade dysplasia is detected and confirmed.

Crohn's disease

Risk of surgery

General risks

Within 10 years of diagnosis, approximately half of all patients will have had an intestinal resection. Of all those having surgery, 40% will have a further operation within 10 years of the first. Resection is more likely for ileal or small bowel disease than for colonic disease.

Risk of surgery for ileocolonic disease

Eighty-seven per cent of patients with ileocolonic Crohn's disease will have at least one operation during the course of their disease. After a resection for ileocolitis the cumulative rate for further surgery is 16% at 5 years and 26% after 10 years.

Risk of surgery for colonic disease

The operation rate for disease confined to the colon is lower because of the smaller risk of obstruction and abscess formation, and because colonic disease is often easier to control with drugs than small bowel disease.

Patients with colonic Crohn's disease have a 40% probability of requiring an operation within 10 years. Breakdown of a primary anastomosis occurs in 17% of patients. The 10-year clinical recurrence rate after a colectomy and ileorectal anastomosis is 65%, and the reoperation rate is 50%.

A stoma has considerably less risk of recurrence than an anastomosis. The clinical, operative and endoscopic recurrence rates for proctocolectomy and ileostomy are approximately half those for ileorectal anastomosis.

Risk of cancer

The risk of colonic cancer in Crohn's disease remains controversial, but it may be increased for patients who have extensive long-standing colonic disease. No surveillance programmes have been undertaken in this condition. However there is an increasing trend to include patients with Crohn's disease in a surveillance programme if they have similar predisposing conditions as patients with ulcerative colitis — long-standing (longer than 8 years) colonic Crohn's disease involving most or all of the colon. There are no data to show benefit from such a surveillance programme in Crohn's disease.

Patients at highest risk of cancer are those with **complicated anorectal disease**, including those with fistulae, strictures, and chronic abscesses. These patients should be kept under review and biopsies taken if the disease changes or appears atypical.

The risk of cancer of the small intestine is much increased in Crohn's disease compared with the general population, but is still a very rare complication. Routine screening is not indicated.

Useful addresses

British Colostomy Association
15 Station Road
Reading
Berkshire
RG1 1LG

British Digestive Foundation
Room D
7 Chandos Street
Cavendish Square
London
W1A 2LN

Ileostomy Association of Great Britain and Ireland
Amblehurst House
Chobham
Woking
Surrey
GU24 8PZ

National Association for Colitis and Crohn's Disease
98a London Road
St Albans
Hertfordshire
AL1 1NX

Index

Page numbers in *italics* refer to the illustrations